Nursing Assessment

Head-to-toe physical assessment in picture

(Health Assessment in Nursing)
2nd Edition

NURSING.com
Jon Haws RN
Sandra Haws RD

Disclaimer

Products produced, published or sold by NURSING.com (the term "NURSING.com" refers collectively to TazKai, LLC, NRSNG, LLC, and NRSNG Academy, LLC and any other D.B.A. of TazKai, LLC) including but not limited to blogs, podcasts, courses, videos, cheatsheets, Scrubcheats™, books, other print and digital materials, and all other products (collectively referred to as the "NURSING.com Products") are for entertainment and informational purposes only and should not be used to make medical diagnosis, give medical advice or prescribe medical treatment.

NURSING.com Products are designed to provide accurate information in regard to the subject matter covered and NURSING.com uses reasonable efforts to ensure such information is accurate. Notwithstanding the foregoing, NURSING.com MAKES NO WARRANTY OR GUARANTY AS TO, AND ASSUMES NO RESPONSIBILITY FOR, THE CORRECTNESS, SUFFICIENCY, ACCURACY OR COMPLETENESS OF INFORMATION OR RECOMMENDATIONS MADE IN NURSING.com PRODUCTS, OR FOR ANY ERRORS, OMISSIONS, OR ANY OUTCOMES RELATED TO YOUR USE OF NURSING.com PRODUCTS.

NURSING.com Products may provide information, guidance, and recommendations related to a variety of subject matters, including but not limited to, medical treatment, emergency care, drugs, medical devices, and side effects; however, research, clinical practice, and government regulations often change the accepted standards and it is SOLELY YOUR RESPONSIBILITY, and not the responsibility of NURSING.com, to determine appropriate medical treatment, the use of any drug in the clinical setting, and for determining FDA status of a drug, reading the package insert, and reviewing prescribing information for the most up-to-date recommendations on dose, precautions, and contraindications, and determining the appropriate usage for a product.

NURSING.com Products were developed based on generally accepted education and nursing principles and standards in the United States, and have not been customized or otherwise specifically designed for use in any other country.

Table of contents

NURSING.com Academy Companion Course

Health Assessment is a critical nursing skill, in fact, we've developed an entire course on Assessments within NURSING.com Academy. NURSING.com Academy helps you master nursing concepts, reduce your study time, and ditch the stress of traditional nursing education. NURSING.com Academy will drastically accelerate the speed at which you master nursing content. As you are reading Health Assessment for Nurses, look at the bottom of the pages for this:

[NURSING.com Academy Lesson: (Lesson Name)]

This is the NURSING.com Academy course and lesson that corresponds to the page you are reading, where you will be able to dive deeper into that specific concept. You can learn more or sign up for the NURSING.com Academy at NURSING.com

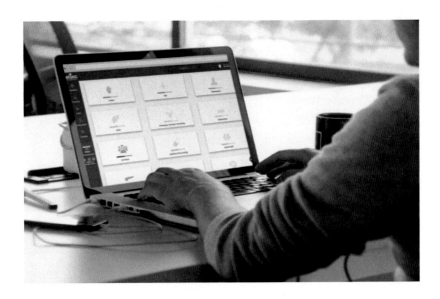

Visit
NURSING.com
to check out our academy lessons!

Head-to-toe Assessment Checklist

General Assessment

Body Structure/Mobility

Behavior

Health History

Vital Signs

Height Weight

Pulse Rate

Respirations

Temperature

Blood Pressure

Pain

Integumentary

Inspect: color, moisture, hair, rashes, lesions, pallor, edema

Palpate: temperature, turgor, lesions, edema, texture

Scalp

Inspect: shape, symmetry

Palpate: tenderness, deformity

Nails

Inspect: shape, color

Palpate: capillary refill

Head

Inspect: symmetry, shape, size, uniformity

Neck

Inspect: symmetry, lesions, scars

Palpate: tenderness, lymph nodes, thyroid gland, TMJ

Eyes

Inspect: interior and exterior, visual fields, acuity, reflexes

Ears

Inspect: color, shape, symmetry, interior inspection

Palpate: tenderness, deformity

Nose

Inspect: shape, symmetry, interior inspection

Palpate: frontal sinus, maxillary sinuses

Mouth and Throat

Inspect: exterior and interior

Thorax and Lungs (anterior and posterior)

Inspection: respiration quality, symmetry, deformity, tracheal location

Palpation: tenderness, fremitus, chest expansion

Percussion: percussive tones, diaphragmatic excursion

Auscultation: breath sounds and quality

Heart and Great Vessels

Inspection: jugular venous pulse

Palpate: pulses, PMI

Auscultate: heart sounds (bell and diaphragm)

Peripheral Vascular System

Inspect: color, edema

Palpate: temperature, edema

Abdomen

Inspect: discomfort, uniformity, color, symmetry, scars, hernia, peristalsis, pulsations

Auscultate: bowel sounds, bruits

Percussion: four quadrants, liver, spleen, renal tenderness

Palpation: light to deep, liver, spleen, aorta, rebound tenderness, fluid wave

Musculoskeletal

Inspection: asymmetry, deformity, atrophy

Palpation: major joints, tenderness, deformity, range of motion

Neurological

Inspect: mental status (health history), cranial nerves, coordination, movement, senses

Palpate: motor strength, muscle tone, reflexes, senses

Genitourinary

Inspect: general appearance, lesions, scars

Palpate: breast exam, testicular exam, prostate exam, vaginal exam, Pap smear

Lymphatic

Palpate: assess lymph node locations

Integumentary

Anatomy

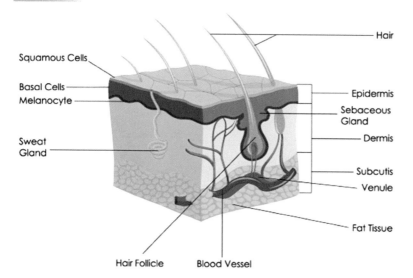

The outermost layer of the skin is called the epidermis. The next layer is the dermis and below that is the subcutaneous layer of fat. Several important glands secrete fluids towards the skin. There are two types of sweat glands. The apocrine sweat glands open into the hair follicles. They respond specifically to emotion or arousal. They begin functioning during puberty. The eccrine sweat glands secrete directly to the skin surface. Their main purpose is the regulation of body temperature. The sebaceous glands secrete a lipid substance into hair follicles.

Hair is a string of proteins that grows from a follicle in the dermis layer of the skin. Hair is made of 3 layers the medulla in the center, the cortex, and then the cuticle.

The nails are made of keratin. The pink color below the nail is due to blood supply to the skin below.

Inspection

Begin your assessment of the skin by looking at the general color or pigmentation of the patient.

The patient's color should be consistent with the genetic makeup of the patient, ranging from pink to dark brown. Darker-skinned people may have areas of lighter pigmentation.

Assess for freckles and birthmarks and use the ABCDE framework to determine abnormality of these markers.

Assess the patient's skin color for any changes in color (also known as pallor), cyanosis, or jaundice. It may be more complicated to notice these changes in darker-skinned individuals. The best place to look for these would be nail beds and lips.

Assess hair growth and pattern. Assess for edema.

Palpation

Palpate the skin and assess the temperature (hypothermia versus hyperthermia). As you feel the skin you should also assess for moisture or diaphoresis.

Assess the mucous membranes for dehydration. The general texture of the skin should be smooth and firm, and thickness of the skin should be uniform throughout the body. The heels and palms may be a little bit thicker.

Assess the skin as well for edema, which is fluid accumulation. You can assess for this by palpating on the skin and seeing if there's an imprint left after you lift your hand up. This is known as pitting edema. It could be graded from a scale of +1 to + 4, with +4 being more severe. Edema can mask other more serious signs and symptoms.

Assess the mobility and turgor of the skin. This can be done by pinching the skin up in a fold, upon releasing the fold it should return back to its normal state.

Assess the skin for vascularity and for bruising or lesions. Document their size, color, elevation, general makeup, as well as the location, and make note of any exudate or odor coming from the lesion.

Abnormal Findings

Cyanosis

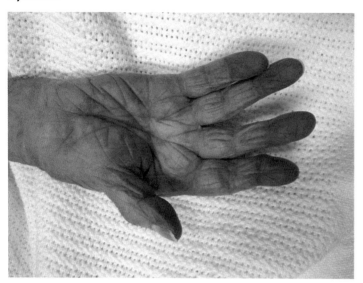

By James Heilman, MD (Own work) [CC BY-SA 3.0 (http://creativecommons.org/licenses/by-sa/3.0)], via Wikimedia Commons

Rash

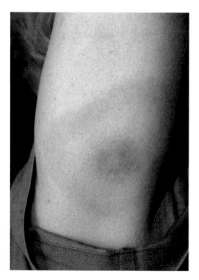

Jaundice

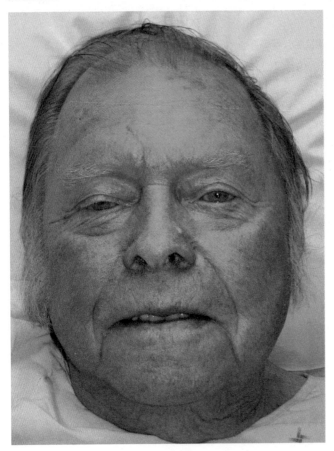

By James Heilman, MD (Own work) [CC BY 3.0 (http://creativecommons.org/
licenses/by/3.0)], via Wikimedia Commons

Macule, Patch, Papule, Plaque, Vesicles, Bulla, Fissure, Erosion, Ulcer

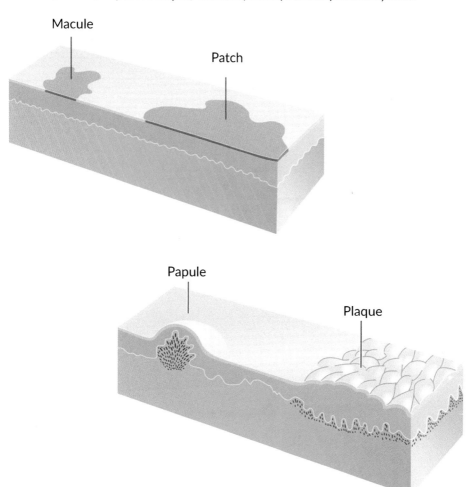

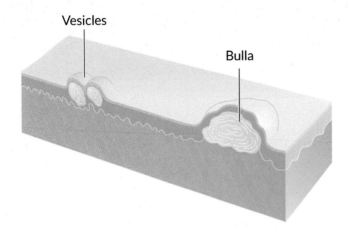

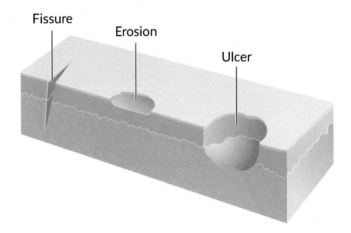

By Madhero88 (Own work) [CC BY-SA 3.0 (http://creativecommons.org/licenses/by- sa/3.0)], via Wikimedia Commons

Scalp

Inspection and Palpation

Inspect and palpate the scalp and hair. Assess for the color of the hair and scalp. Assess for shape and symmetry.

Assess the texture of the hair. This can help with understanding nutritional status. Assess for lesions on the scalp and ensure that the patient's scalp is clean.

Nails

Inspection and Palpation

Inspect and palpate the nails. Assess the shape of the nail as well as the color of the nail beds. They should be smooth, clean and round. Assess the surface of the nail to ensure that it is consistent throughout and that the thickness of the nails are uniform.

Lastly, assess for capillary refill. Press on the nail for a second or two, upon removing pressure, color should return to the nail bed within 1 to 2 seconds. Which indicates normal capillary refill.

Abnormal Findings

Clubbing

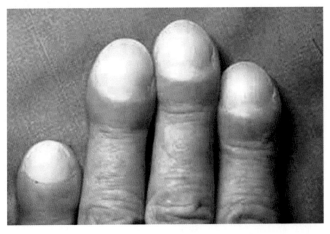

By Desherinka (Own work) [GFDL (http://www.gnu.org/copyleft/fdl.html) or CC BY- SA 4.0-3.0-2.5-2.0-1.0 (http://creativecommons.org/licenses/by-sa/4.0-3.0-2.5-2.0-1.0)], via Wikimedia Commons

[NURSING.com Academy Lesson: Defects of Decreased Pulmonary Blood Flow]

Head

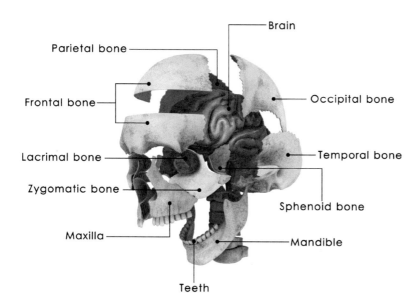

Parietal bone

Brain

Frontal bone

Occipital bone

Lacrimal bone

Temporal bone

Zygomatic bone

Sphenoid bone

Maxilla

Mandible

Teeth

Inspection and Palpation

When assessing the head, start with inspecting and palpating. Inspect the head for general symmetry and appropriate size for the body. The skull should feel symmetrical and smooth. There should be no tenderness on palpation.

Inspect the face for symmetry with the eyebrows, the nose, and the mouth. Make note of any abnormal facial features or swelling or involuntary ticks of the muscles.

Neck

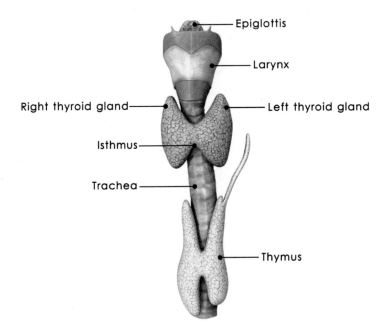

Epiglottis

Larynx

Right thyroid gland

Left thyroid gland

Isthmus

Trachea

Thymus

Inspection and Palpation

Inspect the neck for symmetry and ensure that the neck is midline. Assess for neck range of motion. Is the patient able to point the chin down, lift the chin up, and turn from left to right, as well as the shoulders to the ear and extend the head backward? The motions should be smooth and well-controlled.

Assess for lesions or scars.

Palpate the temporomandibular joint for tenderness.

Palpate the lymph nodes. Use a gentle, circular motion to palpate the lymph nodes in front of the ear and within the neck.

Palpate the thyroid gland.

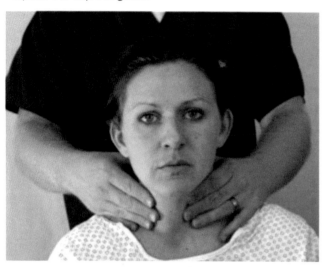

Abnormal Findings

Goiter

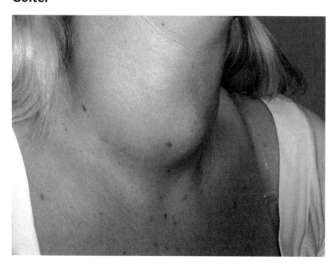

By Drahreg01 (Own work) [GFDL (http://www.gnu.org/copyleft/fdl.html) or CC BY-SA 3.0 (http://creativecommons.org/licenses/by-sa/3.0)], via Wikimedia Commons

Eyes

Anatomy

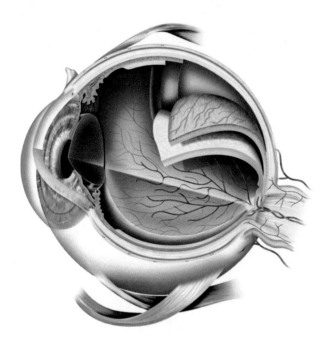

The eye is a sensory organ involved with sight. The eye is protected from external offenses like light or dust by the upper and lower eyelid. The small open space between eyelids is known as the palpebral fissure.

The outermost portion of the eye is the conjuctiva. It lines the inside of the eyelids and the sclera and merges with the cornea which is the outermost covering of the iris and pupil. Behind the cornea is the lens.

A part of the interior of the eye can be visualized with a ophthalmoscope. This area is called the ocular fundus, and in this area the optic disc and macula can be seen.

The eye has three layers: sclera just under the conjunctiva, the choroid in the middle, and the retina on the inside. The retina is where light waves are converted into nerve impulses.

Inspection

When assessing the eyes, inspect the pupils to insure they are equal, round, and reactive to light.

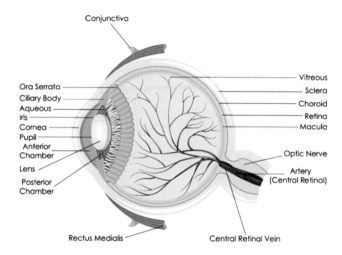

Test for visual acuity with the Snellen chart by having the patient stand 20 feet from the chart. Remove glasses or contact lenses and cover the untested eye.

You should test the visual field. Have the patient look in all directions as you move a pencil in those directions. Eye movement should be fluid and well-controlled.

Inspect extraocular muscle function with the 6 cardinal positions. Move your finger in the 6 positions and have the patient follow with their eyes.

Use the confrontation test to assess visual field. Stand 2 feet away from the patient with a pencil in each hand on either side of the patient. While moving the pencils toward midline have the patient state when they are able to see them.

Assess eyebrows for symmetrical movement bilaterally.

Assess eyelids and lashes, notice any redness, swelling or discharge or lesions.

Assess the general shape of the eye. Inspect the eyeballs for any protrusion or sunken appearance.

Inspect the conjunctiva and the sclera. Ask the patient to look up and while using your thumbs to inspect the conjunctiva and sclera of the patient.

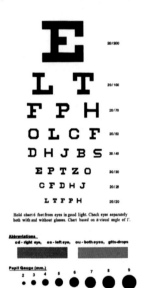

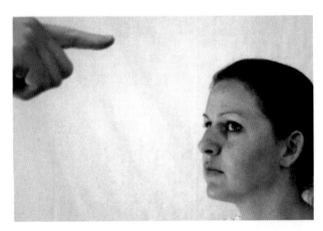

Inspect the interior eyeball structures. Shine a light from side to side and check for smoothness and clarity of the eye.

Inspect the iris, the pupils, and if the pupils are able to accommodate to light. You should determine that both pupils are equal bilaterally. If the patient has 2 different- sized pupils, this is known as anisocoria.

Inspect the ocular fundus by darkening the room and having the patient remove their glasses. Have the patient look at a specific mark with the eyes fixed while the examiner looks into the eyes to inspect the structures of the ocular fundus, specifically the optic disc, retinal vessels, and general background of the macula.

Inspect the color, shape, and margins of the optic disk.

Assess the retinal vessels; the number, the color, and the caliber.

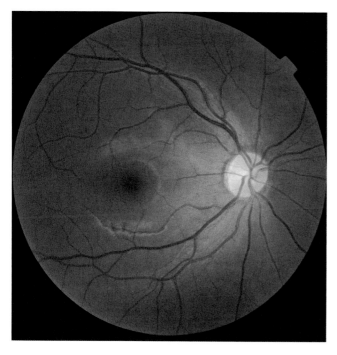

By OptometrusPrime (Fundus Photo, Right Eye (OD) [CC BY-SA 3.0 (https://creativecommons.org/licenses/by-sa/3.0/)]

Abnormal Findings

Pinguecula

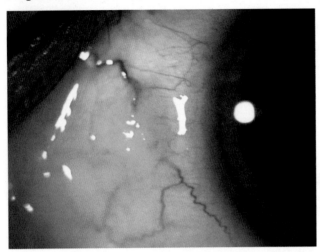

By Red eye2008 (Own work) [CC BY-SA 3.0 (http://creativecommons.org/licenses/
by- sa/3.0) or GFDL (http://www.gnu.org/copyleft/fdl.html)], via Wikimedia Commons

Xanthelasma

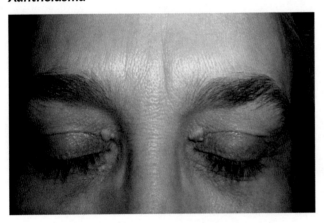

By Klaus D. Peter, Gummersbach, Germany (Own work) [CC BY 3.0 de
(http://creativecommons.org/licenses/by/3.0/de/deed.en)], via Wikimedia Commons

Arcus Senilis

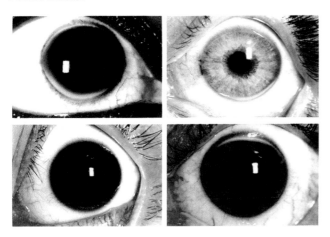

By Loren A Zech Jr and Jeffery M Hoeg [CC BY 2.0 (http://creativecommons.org/licenses/by/2.0)], via Wikimedia Commons

Ptosis

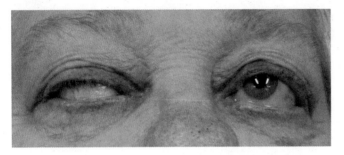

By Loren A Zech Jr and Jeffery M Hoeg [CC BY 2.0 (http://creativecommons.org/
licenses/by/2.0)], via Wikimedia Commons

Exopthalmos

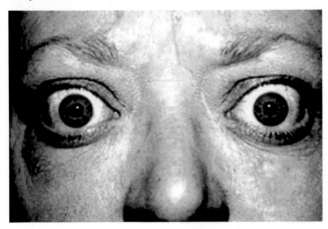

By Jonathan Trobe, M.D. - University of Michigan Kellogg Eye Center (The Eyes Have It)
[CC BY 3.0 (http://creativecommons.org/licenses/by/3.0)], via Wikimedia Commons

Conjunctivitis

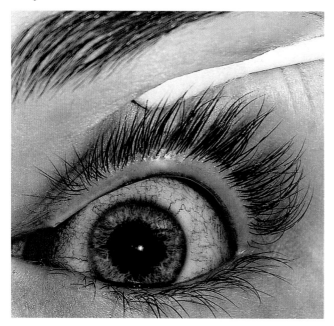

By Joyhill09 [GFDL (http://www.gnu.org/copyleft/fdl.html) or CC BY-SA 3.0 (http://creativecommons.org/licenses/by-sa/3.0)], via Wikimedia Commons

Anisocoria

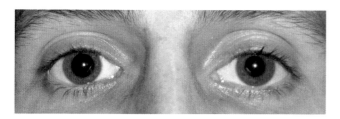

By Russavia (Own Work) [CC BY-SA 3.0 (https://creativecommons.org/licenses/by-sa/3.0/)]

Miosis

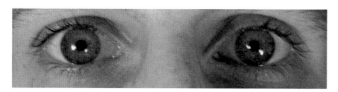

By Anonymous (Anonymous) [CC0], via Wikimedia Commons

Mydriasis

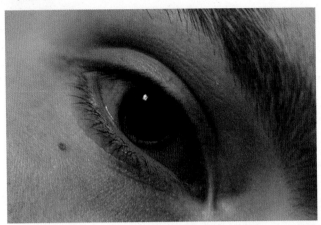

Ears

Anatomy

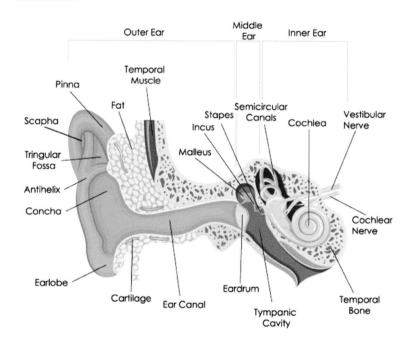

The ears are sensory organs involved with hearing and balance/equilibrium. The ear is divided in to three sections: external ear, middle ear, and inner ear.

The external ear is also known as the pinna or auricle. Sound travels into the external auditory canal and reaches the ear drum or tympanic membrane. This thin membrane separates the external and middle ear.

The ear drum vibrates in response to sound and the vibrations travel through the middle ear. The middle ear contains three small bones called ossicles. They are the incus, malleus, and stapes.

The inner ear contains the bony labyrinth which is an opening in the temporal bone that contains the sensory organs for hearing and equilibrium.

The bony labyrinth has three parts: semicircular canals, vestibule, and cochlea. The cochlea is responsible for turning pressure from sound into impulses that communicate to the brain. The vestibular system is responsible for balance.

Inspection and Palpation

Inspect the general size and shape of the outer ear. They should be equal bilaterally with no obvious swelling or thickening. Assess skin condition; looking for lumps, lesions, or tenderness. Palpating the patient's ear and mastoid process should be painless.

Inspect the external auditory meatus, there should be no swelling or redness. Most patients will have some cerumen, but excessive cerumen would be abnormal.

Inspection of the interior of the ear is called the otoscopic examination. Choose the largest speculum that fits inside the patient's ear comfortably. For adults, pull the pinna up and back. This helps straighten out the ear canal.

Hold the otoscope upside down with the dorsum of your hand along the person's cheek. Inspect the external canal, notice any redness, swelling, discharge, or any foreign bodies within the ear canal.

Assess the tympanic membrane by checking the color and characteristics. It should be translucent with a pearly grey color. The eardrum should be flat and slightly pulled in at the center. The tympanic membrane should be completely intact.

Asses hearing acuity by beginning with the whisper voice test. Stand about 2 feet away and whisper 2 syllable words into the patient's ear while asking them repeat the words they hear.

Assess air and bone conduction with tuning forks. The Webber test involves striking a tuning fork and placing it midline on the patient's skull. The patient should hear the sound equally bilaterally.

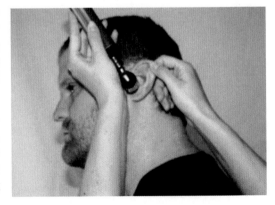

The Rinne test compares air conduction versus bone conduction. Place the tuning fork midline on the patient's skull and ask them to state when they stop hearing the sound.

Abnormal Findings

Ear Drum Retraction

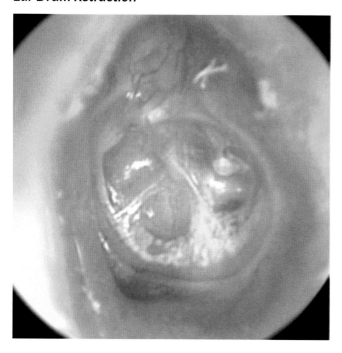

By Adrian L James (Own work) [CC BY-SA 3.0 (http://creativecommons.org/licenses/by-sa/3.0)], via Wikimedia Commons

Otitis Media

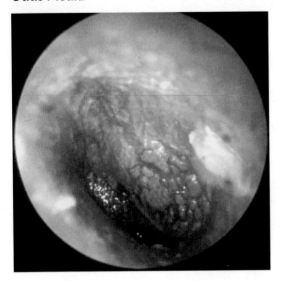

By http://www.sharinginhealth.ca (http://www.sharinginhealth.ca) [CC BY-SA 2.5 (http://creativecommons.org/licenses/by-sa/2.5)], via Wikimedia Commons

Otitis Externa

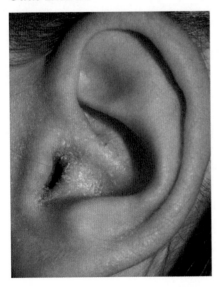

By Klaus D. Peter, Gummersbach, Germany (Own work) [CC BY 3.0 de (http://creativecommons.org/licenses/by/3.0/de/deed.en)], via Wikimedia Commons

Cauliflower Ear

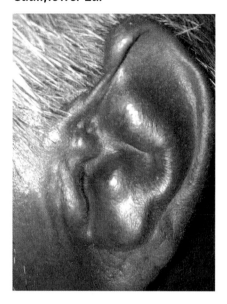

Nose

Anatomy

Inspection and Palpation

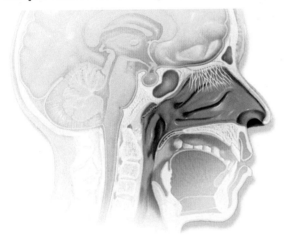

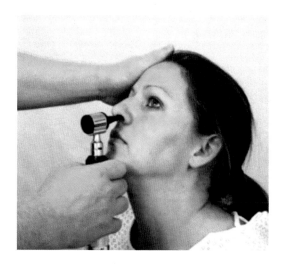

Inspect the nose. It should be symmetric and midline on the face. There should be no deformities or inflammation or skin lesions. Test the patency of the nostrils to reveal any obstruction in the nasal cavity.

Inspect the nasal cavity using an otoscope and a wide-tip speculum. Inspect the nasal mucosa noting its color and assess for any swelling or discharge.

Inspect the two turbinates, the bony ridges coming down the lateral walls of the nose, and also note any polyps or benign growths within the nose.

Palpate the sinus area. You should palpate the frontal sinus, which is directly below the eyebrows, and the maxillary sinus, right below the cheekbones. The patient will feel pressure but they should not feel pain.

Abnormal Findings

Deviated Septum

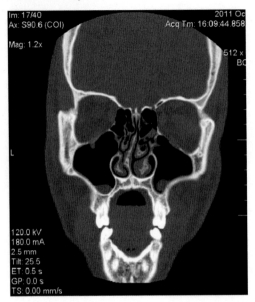

By Mike Gerkin (Own work) [CC BY-SA 3.0 (http://creativecommons.org/
licenses/by- sa/3.0)], via Wikimedia Commons

Nasal Polyp

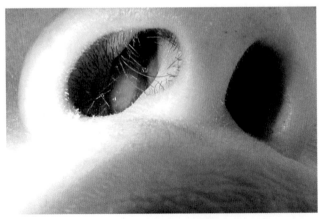

By MathieuMD (Own work) [CC BY-SA 3.0 (http://creativecommons.org/
licenses/by- sa/3.0)], via Wikimedia Commons

Mouth

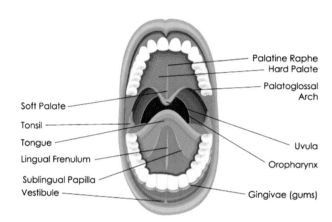

Palatine Raphe
Hard Palate
Palatoglossal Arch
Soft Palate
Tonsil
Tongue
Lingual Frenulum
Sublingual Papilla
Vestibule
Uvula
Oropharynx
Gingivae (gums)

Inspection

Inspect the mouth. Inspect the lips for their color, moisture, and any lesions or discoloration.

Inspect the teeth. The teeth should be straight and evenly spaced. There should not be any absent, loose or abnormally positioned teeth. Ask the patient to bite and note the alignment of the jaw.

Inspect the gums. The gums should look pink. Check for swelling, gingival margins, bleeding, or discoloration.

Inspect the tongue. The tongue should be pink and symmetrical. Some patients may have a thin, white coating on their tongue. To inspect the area beneath the tongue, have the patient touch the roof of their mouth with their tongue. Make note of any ulcerations or nodules.

Inspect the buccal mucosa, which should be soft, pink, and smooth. The Stensen's duct is the opening of the parotid salivary gland.

Inspect the palate. The anterior palate is hard with rugae. The posterior palate is soft. Ask the patient to say "ah" which will cause the soft palate and the uvula to rise which aids in testing cranial nerve X, the vagus nerve.

Abnormal Findings

Cheilitis

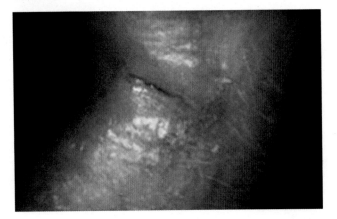

By Lesion (Own work) [CC BY-SA 3.0 (http://creativecommons.org/licenses/by-sa/3.0)], via Wikimedia Commons

Herpes

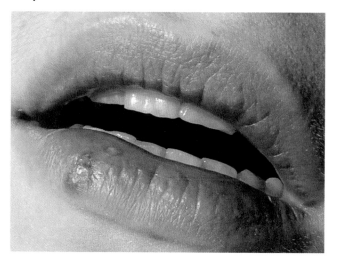

Aphthous Ulcer

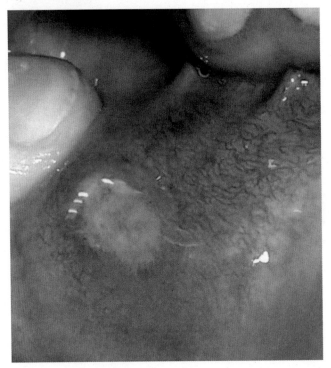

Torus Palantinus

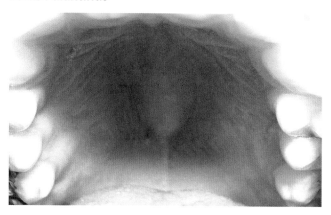

Throat

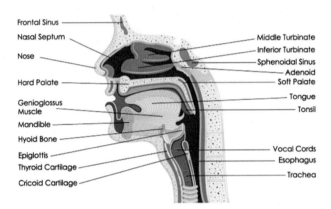

Frontal Sinus
Nasal Septum
Nose
Hard Palate
Genioglossus Muscle
Mandible
Hyoid Bone
Epiglottis
Thyroid Cartilage
Cricoid Cartilage

Middle Turbinate
Inferior Turbinate
Sphenoidal Sinus
Adenoid
Soft Palate
Tongue
Tonsil
Vocal Cords
Esophagus
Trachea

Inspection

Inspect the throat. Inspect the tonsils by having the patient open their mouth. Tonsils are graded on their size with 1+ being visible, 2+ halfway between the tonsillar pillars and uvula, 3+ touching the uvula, and 4+ touching each other. Many patients will have 1+ or 2+ as a normal finding.

- 1+: Visible

- 2+: Halfway between tonsillar pillars and uvula

- 3+: Touching the uvula

- 4+: Touching each other

Inspect the posterior throat for exudate or lesions. Use a tongue blade to elicit a gag reflex. Testing the gag reflex helps with assessing cranial nerves IX and X. Assess cranial nerve XII, (the hypoglossal nerve) by asking the patient to stick their tongue out. The tongue should protrude midline with no deviation from side-to-side.

Tonsillitis

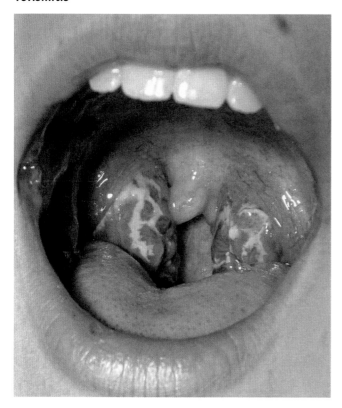

By Nick Berman (Own work) [CC BY-SA 4.0 (http://creativecommons.org/
licenses/by- sa/4.0)], via Wikimedia Commons

Posterior Thorax and Lungs

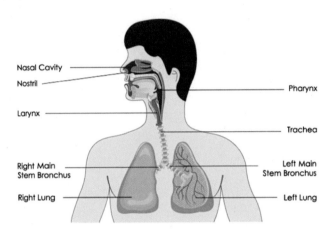

Nasal Cavity
Nostril
Larynx
Right Main Stem Bronchus
Right Lung
Pharynx
Trachea
Left Main Stem Bronchus
Left Lung

Inspection

Inspect the posterior chest, the spine, and spinal process which should be straight and midline. The thorax should be symmetric. The neck and trapezius muscles should be developed normally for the age and lifestyle of the patient. The patient's skin color should be consistent with the patient's background with no abnormal coloring or lesions.

Assess the quality of the patient's breathing.

Palpation

Palpate the posterior chest. Confirm symmetric chest expansion. Place your hands on the posterior chest wall between level T9 and T10. Ask the patient take a deep breath while watching your hands, they should move apart symmetrically.

Palpate for fremitus, which is a palpable vibration. This is done by placing the ball of the fingers on the patients while having them repeat the "ninety-nine". Assess areas of the chest noting that vibration is equal corresponding areas. Fremitus will decrease as you move down.

Palpate the chest wall. Notice any areas of tenderness or decreased temperature or moisture or lesions.

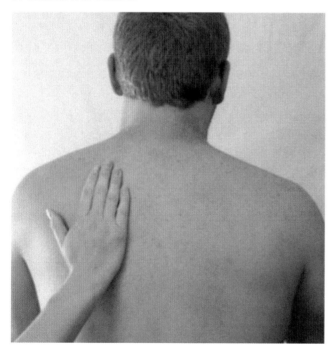

Percussion

Percuss of posterior chest. This is done by starting at the apex and percussing down in the intercostal spaces. Avoid bony processes like the scapula and ribs. Resonance should be heard in healthy lung tissue.

Assess diaphragmatic excursion, which is the movement of the thoracic diaphragm during breathing. This is done by percussing to map out the lower lung border during inspiration and expiration. Normal diaphragmatic excursion should be three to five centimeters.

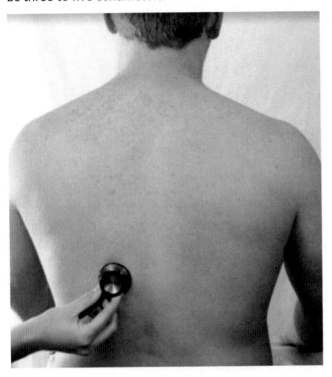

Auscultate

Auscultate the posterior chest. Begin at the apex, around C7 and proceed to the bases around T10. Begin at C7 and move horizontally across the posterior chest. Three types of normal breast sounds will be heard; bronchial, bronchovesicular, and vesicular. Bronchial breath sounds are high pitched and inspiration is shorter than expiration. Bronchovesicular is moderately pitched and inspiration is equal to expiration. Vesicular breath sounds are low pitched and inspiration is longer than expiration. While auscultating breath sounds, be cautious to note any adventitious breath sounds which are abnormal breath sounds.

Anterior Chest

Anatomy

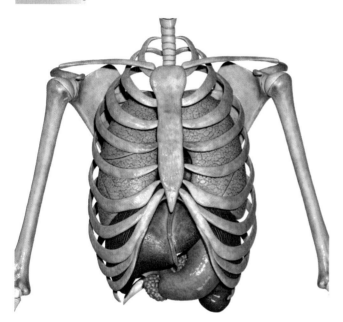

The thorax or chest refers to the area of the body between the neck and abdomen. Within the thorax is the sternum, 12 ribs and 12 thoracic vertebrae.

There are several important anatomical structures in the thorax. The suprasternal notch is a small indentation at the top of the sternum. The manubriosternal angle is where the manubrium joins to the body of the sternum. The costochondral junctions are where the ribs combine with their cartilage. The costal angle is the angle between the right and left costal margin. The zyphoid process protrudes from the bottom of the sternum and this is where the right and left costal margins intersect.

The trachea begins at the cricoid cartilage in the neck and is just in front of the esophagus It splits below the sternal angle into the main bronchi. The bronchi divide into bronchioles which continue to divide. On each bronchiole are alveolar sacs filled with alveoli. The alveoli is where gas exchange occurs.

Inspection

Inspect the shape and configuration of the anterior chest noting that the ribs slope downward and are symmetric, and intercostal spaces are symmetric as well. The patient's abdominal muscles should be appropriately developed for the age and activity level. The patient's face should be relaxed and they should not be showing any signs of tension.

Assess that the trachea is midline.

Assess the patient's skin color, condition, and the quality of respirations. Normal breathing should be relaxed, regular, effortless, and should produce no noise. Assess the patient's respiratory rate and ensure that it is within normal limits.

Percussion

Percuss the anterior chest by beginning at the apex and percussing the intercostal spaces from one side to the other in a descending motion. Dullness is heard over the heart tissue near the fifth intercostal space. In the right midclavicular line, dullness will be heard over the liver. Tympani will be evident over the gastric space.

Auscultation

Auscultate the anterior chest. This is done by beginning at the apex in the supra-clavicular areas and moving down from side-to-side, noting the three types of breath sounds as mentioned earlier; bronchial, bronchovesicular, and vesicular. Listen to one full respiration in each location.

Heart and Great Vessels

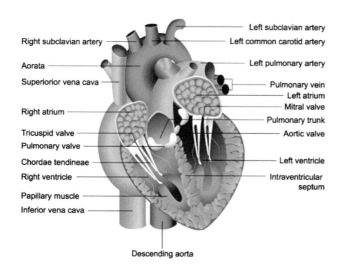

Right subclavian artery
Aorata
Superiorior vena cava
Right atrium
Tricuspid valve
Pulmonary valve
Chordae tendineae
Right ventricle
Papillary muscle
Inferior vena cava

Left subclavian artery
Left common carotid artery
Left pulmonary artery
Pulmonary vein
Left atrium
Mitral valve
Pulmonary trunk
Aortic valve
Left ventricle
Intraventricular septum

Descending aorta

The heart is located in the chest within the rib cage from the 2nd to the 5th inter-costal space and from the right side of the sternum to the midclavicular line.

The top of the heart is called the base and the bottom is the apex. The heart is divided into four chambers: right atrium and ventricle and left atrium and ven-tricle. The atrium holds blood while the ventricle is the strong pumping chamber.

The heart has four valves. There are two semilunar valves between the arteries and ventricles. The right is called the pulmonic valve and the left is called the aor-tic valve. There are two atrioventricular valves between the atria and ventricles. The right is called the tricuspid valve and the left is called the bicuspid or mitral valve. The atrioventricular valves open during diastole (relaxation while the heart is filling with blood). The semilunar valves open during systole (during contraction so blood can be pumped out of the heart).

Heart Sounds S1: closure of the AV valves which is the beginning of systole S2: closure of the SL valves which is the end of systole.

Inspection and Palpation

Palpate the carotid artery. Palpate one artery at a time to avoid compressing blood flow to the brain. Palpate for pulse strength and equality bilaterally.

Auscultate the carotid artery. This is especially indicated in older individuals and those who demonstrate signs of cardiovascular disease. Auscultate for bruit. Listen with the bell of the stethoscope and apply over one carotid artery at a time being cautious not to apply any direct pressure to avoid creating an artificial bruit.

Inspect the jugular venous pulse. This is done by laying the patient at an angle from 30 to 45 degrees to avoid flexing the neck. Ask the patient to turn their head away from the examiner while shining a bright light on the neck. This will highlight the pulsation and shadows of the jugular venous pulse. As a person is raised to the sitting position, the jugular should flatten and disappear usually around 45 degrees.

Inspect the anterior chest for a visible apical impulse. This is also known as point of maximum impulse. If visible, this should be over the fifth intercostal space.

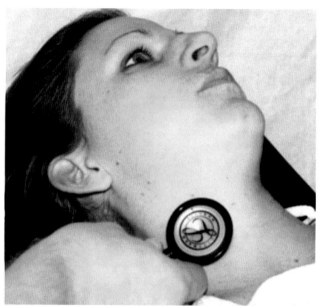

Palpate the apical pulse. This can be done with just one finger pad. Note the location (which should be over the fifth intercostal space), the size, amplitude, and duration. The apical pulse may not be palpable with many patients.

Palpate across the precordium. With the palms of four fingers, palpate gently across the precordium, assessing for any other pulsations.

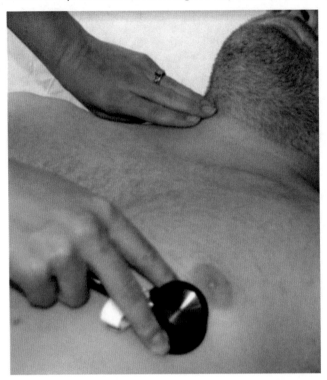

Auscultate

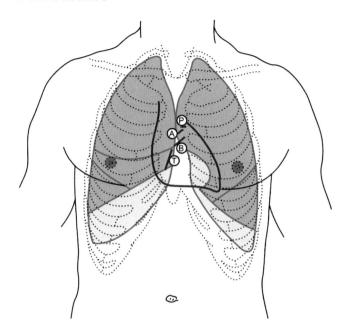

Auscultate the heart sounds. Auscultate the four valve areas. These auscultation areas are not over the anatomical structures, but rather over the areas where sounds are most pronounced and most easily heard. The mnemonic APE To Man is useful in recalling the order of auscultation. APE would stand for aortic, pulmonic, and Erb's point; To Man, tricuspid and mitral.

The aortic valve should be located over the second right intercostal space. The pulmonic valve auscultation area should be located over the second left intercostal space. The tricuspid valve area should be over the left lower sternal border. The mitral valve can be heard over the fifth intercostal space around the left midclavicular line. Actual locations of heart sounds may vary from patient to patient.

Auscultate with the bell for murmurs. Auscultate for any S3 and S4 murmur sounds. Note the rhythm of the heart and the rate. Listen to S1 and S2 separately and listen for any sorts of splitting or murmurs. Murmurs are classified by their timing and loudness (which is graded from grade one through six). Make note of the pitch, quality, location and any radiation of the murmur.

Peripheral Vascular System

Anatomy

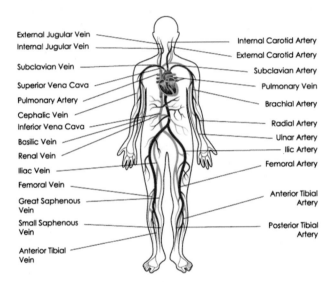

External Jugular Vein
Internal Jugular Vein

Subclavian Vein

Superior Vena Cava

Pulmonary Artery

Cephalic Vein
Inferior Vena Cava

Basilic Vein

Renal Vein

Iliac Vein

Femoral Vein

Great Saphenous Vein

Small Saphenous Vein

Anterior Tibial Vein

Internal Carotid Artery

External Carotid Artery

Subclavian Artery

Pulmonary Vein

Brachial Artery

Radial Artery

Ulnar Artery

Ilic Artery

Femoral Artery

Anterior Tibial Artery

Posterior Tibial Artery

The peripheral vascular system is the transport system in the body. Vessels in the body contain fluids which can carry a variety of substances throughout the body. The heart pumps blood to the lungs where blood picks up oxygen and returns the heart.

The heart then delivers the oxygenated blood and nutrients to the body via arteries. Once oxygen has been picked up by cells in the body, blood and waste travel back to the heart via veins.

Inspection and Palpation

Inspect and palpate the arms. Note the color of the skin and the nail beds, the temperature, texture, and turgor of the skin, and assess for any lesions and edema.

Assess capillary refill. This is done by depressing the nail beds and assessing how long it takes for the color to return. This should happen within one to two seconds.

The arms should be symmetric in size. Assess pulses in all extremities. Palpate radial pulses and dorsalis pedis pulses. Normal would be +2 pulse and they are graded from 0 through +3.

Inspect and palpate the legs. Inspect color, hair growth, venous pattern, and any swelling or lesions. Inspect the hair to see if hair growth is even throughout the legs.

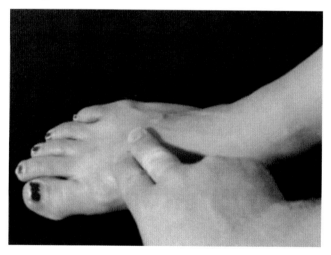

Legs should be symmetric in size without new swelling or atrophy. Assess calf circumference and measure that the widest part is exactly the same on either side.

Palpate to assess the temperature. Palpate the inguinal lymph nodes and note for any unusual size and make sure that they are non-tender.

Palpate peripheral arteries in both legs. The femoral pulse is found just below the inguinal ligament, halfway between the pubis and the anterior-superior iliac spine. Palpate popliteal pulses. This is done with the person's leg extended and relaxed with the examiners fingers just underneath. Posterior tibial pulses are found along the medial malleolus. The dorsalis pedis pulse is lateral and parallel to the big toe.

Doppler may be required to assess these pulses if they are not easily palpated. If doppler is required, mark the location of the pulse with a marker.

Assess for peripheral edema. Edema is graded from 1+ to 4+.

- 1+: being mild pitting and no swelling of the leg
- 2+: moderate: both feet plus lower legs, hands or lower arms
- 3+: severe: generalized bilateral pitting edema, both feet legs, arms, and face
- 4+: very deep pitting and indentation lasts a long time and the leg appears to be very swollen

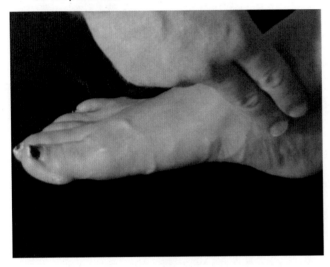

Abnormal Findings

Peripheral Artery Disease (Arterial Ulcer)

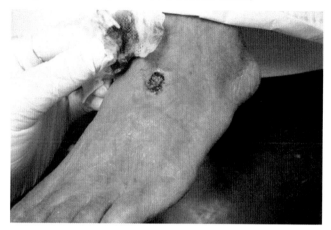

By Jonathan Moore [CC BY 3.0 (http://creativecommons.org/licenses/by/3.0)], via Wikimedia Commons

Chronic Venous Insufficiency

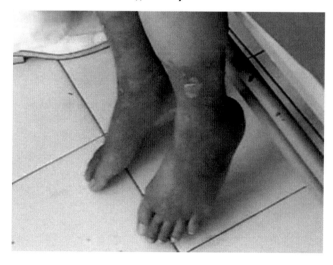

Pitting Edema

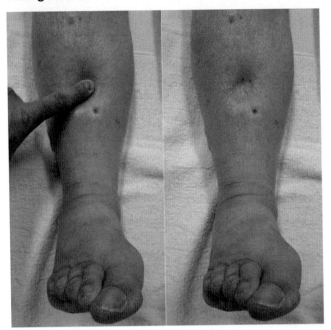

By James Heilman, MD (Own work) [CC BY-SA 3.0 (http://creativecommons.org/
licenses/by-sa/3.0) or GFDL (http://www.gnu.org/copyleft/fdl.html)], via Wikimedia Commons

Abdomen

Anatomy

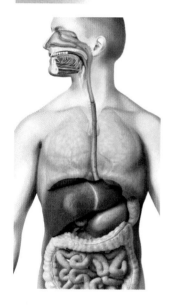

The abdomen is a large cavity below the diaphragm. The largest artery in the abdomen is the aorta which splits into the iliac arteries. The inferior vena cava runs parallel to the aorta and splits into two iliac veins. The liver, pancreas, stomach, appendix, spleen, gallbladder, kidneys, intestines, colon, and reproductive organs are located within the abdomen.

Pancreas: The pancreas is located in the abdomen behind the stomach. It has endocrine functions and exocrine functions. Then pancreas produces important hormones like insulin and glucagon. The pancreas also produces enzymes that help with digestion and absorption of food in the intestines.

Appendix: The appendix is located right where the small intestines join the large intestines. The function of the appendix is unknown, but it can often become inflamed and can sometimes burst.

Stomach: The stomach is an important part of the digestive system. It is located in the upper left quadrant of the abdomen. Food enters the stomach from the esophagus through the lower esophageal sphincter. It mixes with proteases (which breakdown protein) and hydrochloric acid. The stomach muscles thoroughly mix the food to help break it down. Food leaves the stomach through the pyloric sphincter into the intestines.

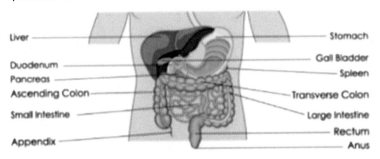

Spleen: The spleen is located in the abdomen just left of the stomach. The spleen helps remove old red blood cells and hold a store of blood. It also synthesizes antibodies.

Small intestines: Once food has been mixed in the stomach, the contents (called chyme) then move into the duodenum of the small intestine. Secretin stimulates the release of bicarbonate, which helps neutralize the acidity of the chyme. Bile from the gallbladder helps emulsify fats and enzymes from the pancreas help break down carbohydrate, fat, and protein. Iron is absorbed in the duodenum. The food then moves into the jejunum where most nutrients are absorbed into the bloodstream. The final segment of the intestines is called the ileum. Vitamin B12 and bile salts are absorbed in the ileum. The intestines contains many small projections, called villi, that significantly increase surface area for absorption of nutrients.

Large intestines: Waste that isn't absorbed in the intestines then travels through the segments of the colon: ascending colon, transverse colon, descending colon; and sigmoid colon. Water is reabsorbed in the colon. Waste then travels through the rectosigmoid junction into the rectum and is excreted via the anal canal.

Kidney: There are two kidneys in the body. They lie on the right and left side of abdomen below the liver and stomach respectively. They sit toward the back of the abdomen. An adrenal gland sits directly above each bean shaped kidney. A renal artery enters the kidney and the renal vein and ureter exit the kidney. The functional unit of the kidney is the nephron. The nephron helps filter out excess water and solutes from the blood. Filtered blood then leaves via the renal vein, and waste via the ureter.

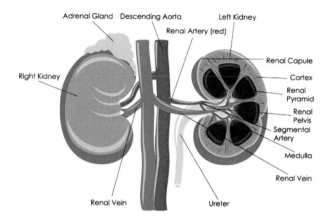

The kidneys play many vital roles in the body including removal of waste products, regulation of blood pressure and electrolytes, acid-base balance reabsorption of amino acids, glucose, and water, hormone production of calcitriol and erythropoietin, and enzyme production of renin.

Liver: The liver is located in the upper right quadrant of the abdomen. The liver has two lobes and sits protected below the ribs. Once blood has picked up nutrients from the intestines, its first stop is the liver. The liver removes chemicals and breaks down drugs.

The liver produces bile which is secreted into the intestines to aid in the absorption of fat. It can synthesize glucose, amino acids, proteins, cholesterol, and triglycerides. It also produce clotting factors. The liver stores glycogen (carbohydrate) and fat soluble vitamins, converts ammonia into urea, and conjugates bilirubin for excretion. This is not an all inclusive list, just an overview of some of the liver's most important functions.

Gallbladder: The Gallbladder is located under the liver. Once the liver produces bile, it travels to the gallbladder for storage. When a meal is ingested, the gallbladder can release the stored bile into the intestines to aid in the absorption of fats.

Inspection

Inspect the contour of the abdomen. This is done by stooping to view across the abdomen to determine if it is flat to slightly rounded. Assess the symmetry of the abdomen by shining a light across and assessing for any bulging, visible masses, or asymmetry.

Assess the umbilicus and notice any discoloration, inflammation, or hernia. There should be none.

Assess the skin texture and color. There should be no lesions or scars. If scars are present note the length and general nature.

Assess for any pulsations or movement in the abdominal area. In some individuals, it may be possible to see pulsations of the aorta. Respiratory movements may also be seen in patients.

Peristalsis may be visible in some patients.

Auscultate

Auscultation comes after inspection in the abdomen so that palpation does not disrupt bowel sounds and change your assessment.

Begin in the right lower quadrant, and use the diaphragm of the stethoscope pressed lightly against the skin. Note bowel sound characteristics and frequency. They should be anywhere from 5 to 30 times per minute.

It is not necessary to count bowel sounds, but note if they are hypoactive, hyperactive or normal. Listen for one full minute in each abdominal quadrant to determine activity.

Auscultate vascular sounds within the abdomen. You should listen for any bruits. You're going to be listening to the aorta, the left renal artery, the iliac artery, and the femoral artery. You may need to use firmer pressure to listen for these sounds.

Percussion

Percuss for tympany. Percuss to determine the location and size of the liver and the spleen. Percuss in all four quadrants. Tympany will be heard due to air in the intestines. A duller sound would indicate a mass, distended bladder, or adipose tissue.

To measure the size of the liver, begin in the right midclavicular line. Percuss down the right midclavicular line, listening for when lung resonance stops; The sound will change to a dull sound. Mark that spot, which should be around the fifth intercostal space. Continue percussion until tympany is heard once again. This indicates the lower border of the liver.

Measure the distance between the two marks. This indicates the size of the liver. It should range from 6 to 12 centimeters in healthy adults.

To assess the spleen begin by percussing a dull tone over the ninth to eleventh intercostal space, on the left midaxillary line.

Percussion of the kidneys aids in assessment of pain and tenderness. This is done by placing the nondominant hand over the costovertebral angle. The nondominant hand is struck with the ulnar surface of the dominant hand made into a fist. Repeat over both kidneys.

Palpation

Begin palpation by working from light to deep palpation. You begin with light palpation with the forefingers close together, and you should make a small circular motion. Lift the fingers between the quadrants. As you're moving around the patient, you should assess for any guarding and notice if the patient is feeling pain.

Upon completion of light palpation, move on to deep palpation. To do this place hands one on top of the other, the top hand pushes the bottom hand. As this is done, take note of the location size and consistency of the abdomen, as well as any tenderness.

Assess for the colon, there may be some tenderness over the colon which is a normal finding. If a mass is felt note the location, size, consistency, and any tenderness.

Assess the location of the liver, via palpation. Place your left hand under the person's back, and lift up to support the abdominal contents. You should then place your right hand on the right upper quadrant, and push deeply down and under the right costal margin. The person should take a deep breath, and with this you should be able to feel the edge of the liver. The liver may not be palpable.

The spleen generally is not palpable. If it is palpable, it may be due to being enlarged. Reach your left hand over the abdomen, and behind the left side of the eleventh and twelfth ribs. You should then place your right hand on the left upper quadrant, with the right fingers pointing towards the left axilla. Push your hand deeply down under the left costal margin. Ask the person to take a deep breath.

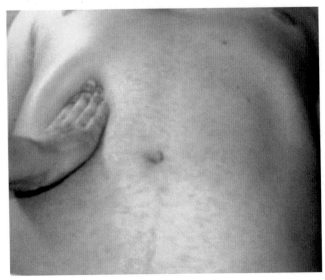

When assessing the kidneys place your hands together and position them at the person's right flank, and then press firmly and deeply, and ask the person to take a deep breath. You should feel no change. You may feel the lower portion of the kidney. Do the same thing on the left side, with the left kidney sitting about one centimeter higher than the right kidney. It should not normally be palpable.

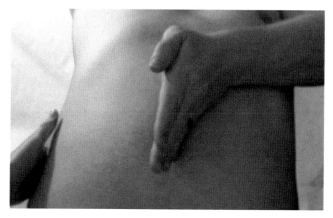

Palpate the aorta, use your thumbs to palpate the aortic pulsation in the upper abdomen. Assess for costovertebral angle tenderness. Place one hand at the costovertebral angle, and the person should feel no pain.

Assess for rebound tenderness to identify peritoneal irritation. To do this hold your hand perpendicular to the abdomen, and push down gently, slowly and deeply, then lift up quickly. If the patient feels rebound tenderness, this is a sign of peritoneal inflammation. Ask where the pain is most intense.

If the patient has a distended abdomen, testing for a fluid wave will help to distinguish between dilated loops of bowel, fat, and free fluid. Have the patient place the ulnar edge of their hand in the umbilical area, mid-line abdomen. You should then place your left hand on the person's right flank, and with your right hand reach across the abdomen and give the left flank a firm shake. If ascites is present, this will generate a fluid wave through the abdomen. A distinct tap on your opposite hand if ascites is present.

Abnormal Findings

Ascites

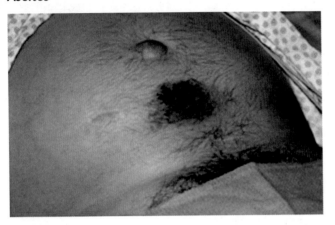

Cullen's Sign

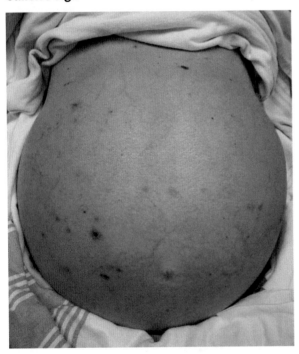

By Herbert L. Fred, MD and Hendrik A. van Dijk (http://cnx.org/content/m14904/latest/) [CC BY 2.0 (http://creativecommons.org/licenses/by/2.0)], via Wikimedia Commons

Musculoskeletal

Anatomy

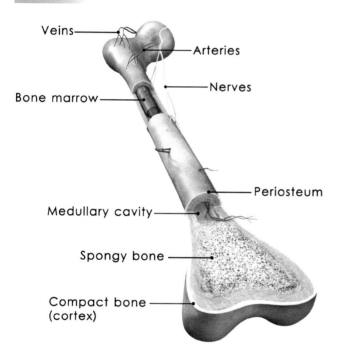

Veins
Arteries
Nerves
Bone marrow
Periosteum
Medullary cavity
Spongy bone
Compact bone (cortex)

The musculoskeletal system is comprised of bones, joints and muscles. The bones provide support and protection for vital organs in the body. Bones also store minerals like phosphorus and calcium and produce red and white blood cells.

Bones are connected by joints. Synovial joints contain a cavity filled with synovial fluid. Cartilage covers each bone at the joint and ligaments connect the two bones and help strengthen the joint. In certain areas of the body there are fluid filled sacs called bursa that help at points of possible friction (prepatellar bursa of the knee).

Muscles attach to bone via tendons. Muscles are made of actin and myosin filaments that allow for movement via contraction or relaxation of the muscle fibers. There are three different types of muscle; skeletal, smooth, and cardiac.

Skeletal muscle is a voluntary muscle. It is connected to our skeleton via tendons and is involved in movement. Smooth muscle is involuntary and is found within organs of the body. Cardiac muscle is involuntary. It is similar to skeletal muscle, but found in the heart.

Inspection and Palpation

When assessing the musculoskeletal system, begin with inspection. Inspect corresponding joints, structure, and function of each joint to determine if full range of motion is present. Note the size of each joint, color, swelling, and any masses or deformity on the joint. Palpate the joint and skin to note temperature, musculoskeletal or muscular deformations, or swelling at the joints.

Assess range of motion of the joints by asking the patient to do active range of motion in the joint corresponding to the type of joint that it is (flexion, extension, abduction, adduction, pronation, supination, circumduction, elevation, depression, rotation, protraction, retraction, eversion, and inversion). Have the patient attempt these movements in each of their joints.

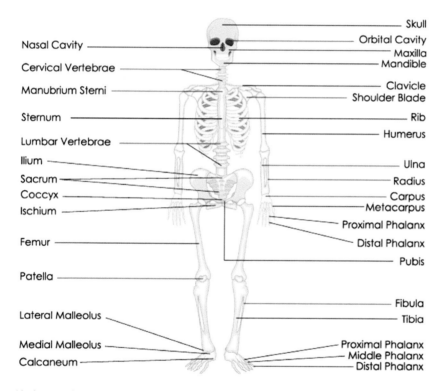

If the patient is unable to do so, attempt passive range of motion. Assist the patient with passive range of motion. If they are unable to complete passive range of motion exercises, do not force any movements. You can use a goniometer to measure the angles at which the patient is able to move. Joint motion should not cause pain or tenderness, or crepitation.

Assess the cervical spine. Inspect the spine first to see that it is aligned with the head and neck, and that it is centered. Palpate the spine and spinal processes. They should feel firm with no spasms or tenderness.

Ask the patient to touch chin to chest and lift their chin toward the ceiling. Touch each ear toward the corresponding shoulder without lifting the shoulder and turn the chin toward each shoulder. The patient should be able to do these movements equally bilaterally, without any sort of pain.

Assess the upper extremities. Inspect both shoulders, posterior and anteriorly assessing the size, and check for any atrophy, deformity or swelling. Palpate the shoulders and assess that there are no spasms, tenderness, swelling or heat.

To test range of motion in the upper extremities ask patient stand with arms at sides and elbows extended. Have the patient move each arm forward in upward arcs and vertical arcs. They should then rotate the arms internally, behind the back, and place back of hands as high as possible.

Test the strength of the shoulder by asking the person to shrug the shoulders up and place a slight amount of resistance.

Inspect the elbow, inspect the size and contour, notice any sorts of deformity, swelling, or lesions. Test range of motion by asking the person to bend and straighten the elbow.

Inspect the wrist and hand, noting position, contour and shape. The fingers should lie straight along the same axis as the forearm. There should be no swelling, redness or deformity. The skin should be smooth, the muscle should be full. You should palpate each joint in the wrists and hands.

There should be no bogginess. The surfaces should be smooth. Test range of motion on the wrists and hands by having the patient bend the hand up at the wrist, bend the hand down, and bend the fingers up and down. The patient should be able to have their palms flat, and turn them inward and outward, spread the fingers apart and make a fist, and touch the thumb to each finger on the hand.

Assess the lower extremities. Begin by assessing the hip and the hip joint. Assess that there is symmetry at the level of the iliac crest, and that the patient has a smooth gait.

Lay the patient in a supine position and palpate the hip joints to test for range of motion in the hip. Have the patient raise each leg with knee extended, and bend each knee up to the chest while keeping the other leg straight. The patient should be able to swing the leg laterally then medially with the knee straight. The patient should be able to, in a standing position, swing a straight leg back behind the body

Next, inspect the knee. Inspect the lower ligament, the knee shape, and contour. There should be no swelling within the knee. Check the quadricep muscle and anterior thigh for any atrophy. Assess range of motion by asking the patient to bend and extend each knee. Have the patient walk. Assess ambulation as well as range of motion during ambulation.

Assess strength by asking the person to keep the knee flexed while applying a slight amount of pressure.

Inspect the ankle and foot. Compare both feet, the positions of toes, and characteristics. Assess for any abnormalities.

Assess the spine. The person should be standing. Place yourself far enough back so that you can see the entire back. Note if the spine is straight by following an imaginary vertical line from head, through the spinous processes and down to the gluteal cleft.

The person's knees should be aligned with the trunk and should be pointing forward. From the side, you should note a normal convex thoracic curve and a concave lumbar curve. You should assess range of motion of the spine by asking the person to bend forward and touch the toes. They should be able to do this in a smooth fashion.

Assess for Homans sign to identify DVT.

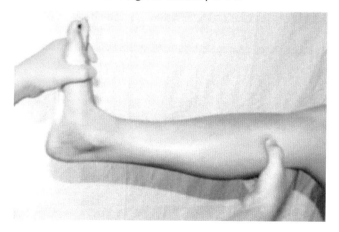

Abnormal Findings

Kyphosis

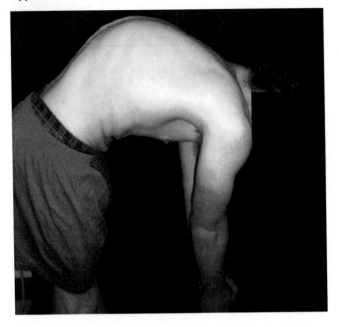

By MusicNewz (Own work this is me) [CC0], via Wikimedia Commons

Scoliosis

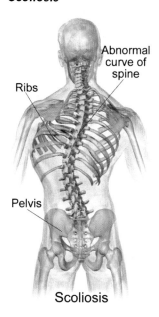

Abnormal curve of spine

Ribs

Pelvis

Scoliosis

Kyphosis, Lordosis

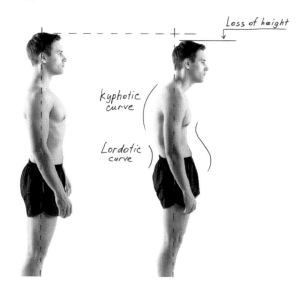

Loss of height

Kyphotic curve

Lordotic curve

Neurological

Anatomy

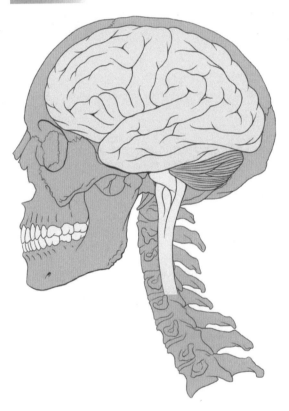

By Patrick J. Lynch, medical illustrator - Patrick J. Lynch, medical illustrator, CC BY 2.5, https://commons.wikimedia.org/w/index.php?curid=1496706

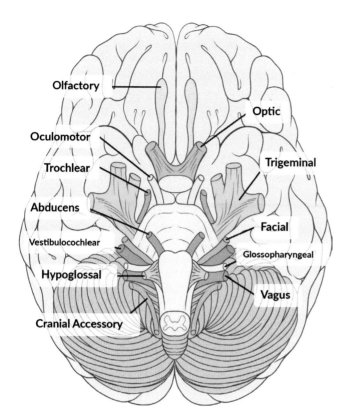

Olfactory

Optic

Oculomotor

Trochlear

Trigeminal

Abducens

Facial

Vestibulocochlear

Glossopharyngeal

Hypoglossal

Vagus

Cranial Accessory

The central nervous system (CNS) is composed of the brain and spinal column. The brain is encased by the skull and the spinal column by the vertebrae. The primary cell of the CNS is the neuron which has unique capabilities. The brain consists of a right and left hemisphere connected by a group of nerves called the corpus callosum. Each hemisphere contains a frontal lobe, temporal lobe, parietal lobe, and occipital lobe.

In the middle of the brain is the thalamus. It relays sensory signals to the cerebral cortex. It is also involved in sleep wake cycles.

The hypothalamus located just below the thalamus plays a role in hunger, thirst, sleep, emotions, temperature, and stimulation of the pituitary.

Posterior to the hypothalamus is the midbrain and below that is the pons. They are involved in motor and sensory functions.

The cerebellum is associated with balance, equilibrium, coordination, and muscle tone. The medulla helps regulate respiratory, gastrointestinal, and heart functions.

There are 12 pairs of cranial nerves and 31 pairs of spinal nerves. The cranial nerves originate in the brain while the spinal nerves originate from different sections of the spinal cord. The spinal nerves are further classified based on location: sacral spinal nerves, thoracic spinal nerves, etc.

Neurons are the primary cell found in the central nervous system. They have a unique shape that allows them to be quick and efficient communicators. This allows us to instantly sense pain in our hand from a hot stove.

Neurons are capable of transmitting electric impulse as well as communicating chemically via neurotransmitters.

Level of Consciousness

When conducting the neurological system assessment, begin by assessing level of consciousness. Is the person alert, awake, and aware of the stimulus in their environment? Are they oriented to person, time, situation, and place? What's their facial expression? What is the quality of their speech? What is their general mood and affect?

Assess the appearance of the patient, position, posture, dress and grooming.

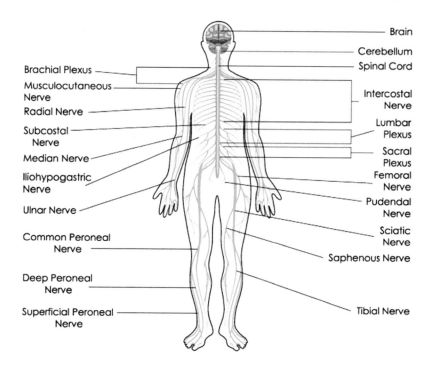

Assess cognitive function. Is the person oriented to time, place, and person? Assess attention span. Are they able to focus on the interview? Are they able to focus on you and what is being done at the moment? What is their recent memory? Are they able to recall why they're in the hospital, what happened, and what brought them to the hospital?

Assess remote memory, past events, and birth dates. What is their judgment? Assess thought processes. Is the person making sense? Are they able to make sense of what is happening? Assess their perceptions, ask them questions about their perception of the world.

Screen them for suicidal thoughts. Ask if they have any thoughts of hurting themselves.

Further assess neurological status. Are they alert? Meaning, are they awake and readily aroused? Are they fully aware of what's happening? Are they lethargic or somnolent, not fully alert, drift into sleep, or requiring stimulation? Are they obtunded, sleeping most of the time, or very difficult to arouse? Are they in a stupor, responding only to vigorous shaking?

Are they in a coma, completely unconscious? Each institution might have different definitions and states for level of consciousness, so it is important to understand how your hospital and your organization determines level of consciousness.

Test cranial nerves. Test cranial nerve II the (optic nerve) by testing visual acuity. Assess cranial nerves II, IV, and VI, (ocular motor, trochlear and abducens nerves). Assess pupil size, regularity, equality, and reaction to light. Are they equally round and reactive to light? This is known as PERRLA (Pupils Equal Round Reactive to Light). Assess for extra ocular movements by assessing for the six cardinal positions.

Assess cranial nerve V (the trigeminal nerve) by assessing motor function. Palpate the temporal masseter muscles as the person clenches their teeth. With the person's eyes closed, test light touch sensation by touching the forehead, cheeks and chin, and having the person state when they feel that they're being touched.

Test the facial nerve (cranial nerve VII) by motor function. Note facial symmetry as the person responds, as they smile, frown, close eyes tightly, and lift eyebrows to show teeth. Assess for symmetry on each side.

Olfactory-Sensory Optic-Sensory Oculomotor-Motor Trochlear-Motor Trigeminal-Both Abducens-Motor Facial-Both Vestibulocochlear-Sensory Glossopharyngeal-Both Vagus-Both Accessory-Motor Hypoglossal-Motor

Inspect and palpate the motor system. Assess cerebellar function by assessing gait and balance. Is the person able to walk in a smooth gait, and is it rhythmic, effortless, and coordinated? Use the Romberg test by asking the person to stand up with their feet together. Have the person stand with their feet together and close their eyes, are they able to stand in a completely balanced and coordinated fashion for 20 seconds?

Assess the sensory system. The person needs to be alert, comfortable and cooperative in order to do this. Assess for superficial pain by using something sharp and something dull to touch the patient. Determine if the patient is able to distinguish between sharp and dull.

Assess stereognosis by placing different objects in the patient's hand with their eyes closed, and determine if they can distinguish between items like paperclips, keys, and coins.

Assess reflexes. Reflexes are graded from zero to four: zero, no response, to four plus, very brisk, hyperactive.

- 0: no response
- 1+: diminished
- 2+: average or normal
- 3+: brisker than average
- 4+: very brisk, hyperactive, clonus, indicative of disease.

Assess the bicep reflex, which will test C5 and C6.

Assess the tricep reflex, which would be C7 and C8.

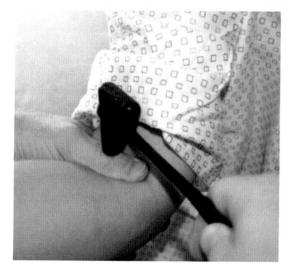

Assess patellar reflex, L2 to L4. The achilles reflex tests L5 to S2.

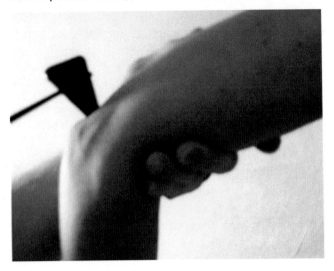

Assess achilles reflex.

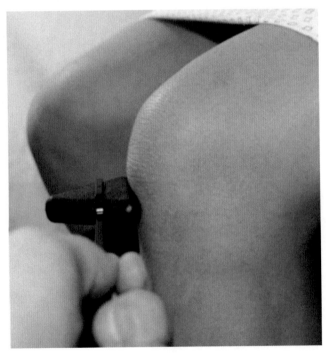

Assess for Babinski reflex by drawing a light stroke from the person's heel to the person's toes in the shape of a J. The normal response is the plantar flexion of the toes, which would be bringing the toes forward toward the stimulus. A positive Babinski reflex would indicate upper motor neuron disease.

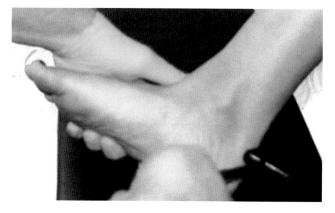

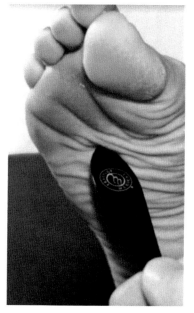
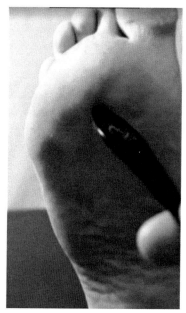

Abnormal Findings

Bells Palsy

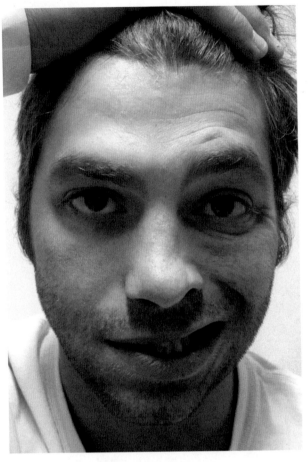

By James Heilman, MD (Own work) [CC BY-SA 3.0 (http://creativecommons.org/licenses/by-sa/3.0) or GFDL (http://www.gnu.org/copyleft/fdl.html)], via Wikimedia Commons

Dystonia

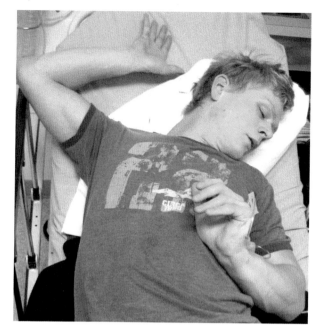

By James Heilman, MD (Own work) [CC BY-SA 3.0 (http://creativecommons.org/licenses/by-sa/3.0) or GFDL (http://www.gnu.org/copyleft/fdl.html)], via Wikimedia Commons

Meningitis (neck stiffness)

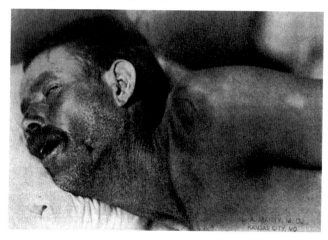

Positive Babinski Sign

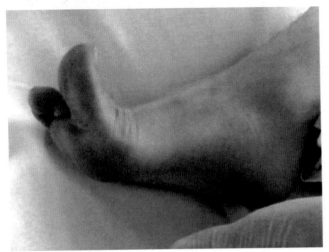

Male Genitourinary

Anatomy

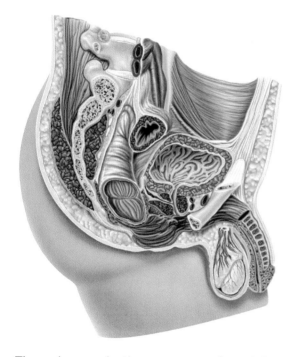

The male reproductive system consists of the scrotum, penis, testis, epidydimis, and vas deferens. The urethra runs through the center of the penis and ends at the tip where waste is removed. The scrotum is a loose sac behind the penis that holds the testis.

Above the testis lie the epididymis which stores sperm that is produced in the testes. The epididymis combines with the vas deferens. The vas deferens with several other vessels is called the spermatic cord.

Puberty typically begins between 9 1/2 and 13 1/3 years of age.

The prostate is found in males, located just below the bladder. It secretes and alkaline fluid that helps maintain sperm viability. It is divided into two lobes by a groove called the median sulcus. Two glands called seminal vesicles secrete a fluid that has fructose to feed the sperm.

Inspection and Palpation

Inspect and palpate the scrotum. Scrotal size will vary depending on patient and room temperature. Asymmetry is normal with the left scrotal half lower than the right. There should be no lesions or cysts.

Palpate each half between your thumb and first two fingers. Testis should feel oval. They should be freely movable and slightly tender. There should be no other scrotal content.

Inspect and palpate for hernia by inspecting the inguinal region for bulge. Palpate the inguinal canal while the patient strains down. Inspect here for inguinal lymph nodes by palpating along the vertical chain within the upper inner thigh.

Instruct the patient to conduct a testicular self-examination once a month, the best time for this being after a warm shower.

Prostate Examination

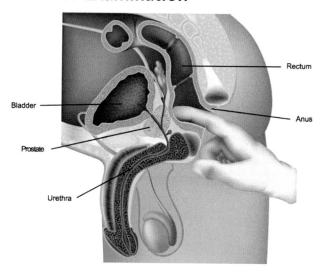

Palpate the prostate gland by pressing into the gland to note the size. The size should be about two-and-a-half centimeters long, about four centimeters wide and should not protrude more than one centimeter into the rectum. Its shape should be heart shape and the surface should be smooth. It should be elastic, rubbery, and slightly movable. There should be no tenderness on palpation. As the examination finger is withdrawn assess any signs of bright blood or mucous on the glove. At this time test stool for occult blood.

Female Genitourinary

Anatomy

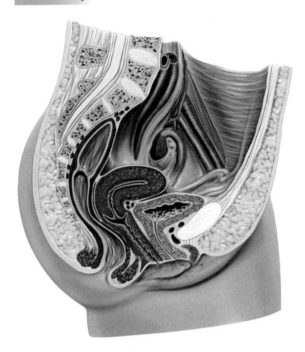

The female reproductive system includes the breasts, vulva, mons pubis, vestibule, clitoris, vagina, cervix, uterus, ovaries, and fallopian tubes.

The mons pubis is a pad of adipose tissue and covers the symphysis pubis. The vestibule is surrounded by the labia minora and labia majora. It includes the urethral meatus and vaginal opening.

The clitoris is located anterior to the urethral meatus which is anterior to the vaginal opening. Two bartholin's glands sit next to the vaginal opening and secret mucus during intercourse. The vagina extends up into the pelvis and ends at the uterine cervix.

Two fallopian tubes extend from the top of the uterus up near the ovaries. Ovaries develop ova or eggs and produce hormones.

Puberty in girls starts between 8 1/2 and 13 years of age. Signs include breast growth, and pubic hair growth, and menarche.

The primary function of the female breast is milk production after childbirth. The breasts lie above the pectoralis muscle between rib 2 and 6.

The axillary Tail of Spence is where a small section of breast tissue extends up into the axilla. The breast is made predominantly of adipose tissue, with some glandular tissue and 4 lactiferous ducts that lead toward the nipple.

The breast tissue is held in place by Cooper's ligaments that connect to chest muscle. The breast is divided into 4 sections: upper outer, lower outer, upper inner, lower inner. The central axillary nodes, pectoral nodes, subscapular nodes, and lateral nodes of the lymphatic system all provide drainage from the breast.

Inspection and Palpation

When conducting the assessment of the female genitourinary system, you should note skin color, and hair distribution.

The labia majora should be symmetrical and well-formed. There should be no lesions or cysts. With gloved hands, separate the labia majora to inspect the clitoris. The labia minora should be dark pink, moist, and symmetric. The perineum should be smooth while the anus has coarse skin with increase pigmentation.

Palpate the clitoral gland. Assess the urethra and Skene's gland. Insert your finger into the vagina and apply pressure up and out. There should be no pain upon doing this.

Assess the Bartholin's gland by palpating the posterior part of the labia majora.

Inspect the genitalia by using a speculum for examination. With the speculum inserted, inspect the cervix. The color should be pink and even within a female who is not pregnant. The position should be midline. The size is about two-and-a-half centimeters. The os is small and round in women who have never been pregnant. In parous women, it is a horizontal, irregular slit. It should be smooth.

If there are secretions depending on menstrual cycle, they should be odorless.

Obtain cervical cultures (Pap smear or Papanicolaou smear) to screen for cervical cancer.

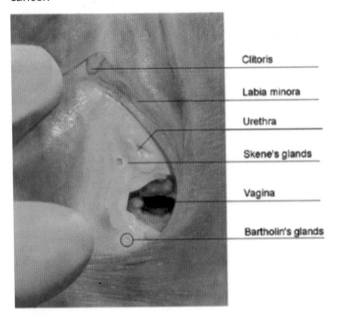

Clitoris

Labia minora

Urethra

Skene's glands

Vagina

Bartholin's glands

Bimanual Examination

With the woman in a lithotomy position, one hand will be placed on the abdomen. With the other hand insert two fingers into the vagina. Palpate the vaginal wall. It should be smooth with no areas of induration or tenderness. It should feel consistent throughout and be evenly rounded, with the cervix able to move from side-to-side.

With the abdominal hand, push the pelvic organs closer to your intervaginal fingers to palpate. Palpate the uterine wall. It normally feels firm and smooth. The uterus should be moved freely and non tender.

Conduct a recto-vaginal examination to assess the recto- vaginal septum, posterior uterine wall, cul-de-sac, and rectum. This may feel uncomfortable to the woman and feel as though she were having a bowel movement. With one hand, insert one finger into the anus and one into the vagina, and with the other hand to apply pressure to the abdomen.

The recto-vaginal septum should feel smooth and thin. The uterine wall and fundus should feel firm and smooth. As rectal finger is withdrawn assess for any signs of blood.

Breasts and Axilla

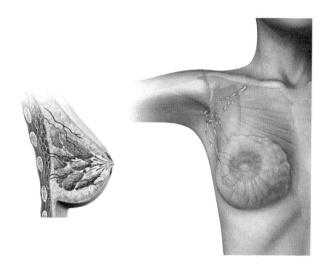

Inspection and Palpation

Inspect the breast. Note asymmetry and size. There may be a slight amount of asymmetry in the size of the breasts which is normal. The skin should be smooth. There should be no lesions, or dimpling, or redness. There should be no edema.

There should be no bulging, discoloration, or edema in lymphatic draining areas. The nipples should be symmetrically located and should usually protrude, although some may be flat or inverted. If an inverted nipple is noted, question the patient if that is new occurrence or preexisting.

Assess for retraction by asking the woman to lift both arms above her head, both breasts should move up symmetrically. Ask the patient to place her hands on her hips and push her two palms together. There will be slight lifting of both breasts.

Inspect and palpate the axilla. Inspect the skin for any rash or infection. Lift the patient's arm and support it yourself so that her muscles relax. Reach your fingers into the axilla and move them firmly down in each direction. The lymph nodes are generally not palpable and there should be no tenderness when you palpate.

Palpate the breast. Ask the patient to lay in a supine position with a small pad under the side to be palpated. Use the pads of your first three fingers and make a gentle rotation movement on the breast. Palpate from the nipple and move outward, feeling for any nodules. Make note of any discharge.

Note the location, size, shape, consistency, skin color, and tenderness of any lumps or masses.

Instruct the patient to conduct a breast self-examination (BSE). The best time for this is right after the menstrual period or the fourth through seventh day of the menstrual cycle.

When assessing the male breast, inspect it and note any lumps or swelling. Gynecomastia is enlargement of the breast tissue. There should be no nodules or swelling in the male breast.

Lymphatic System

Anatomy

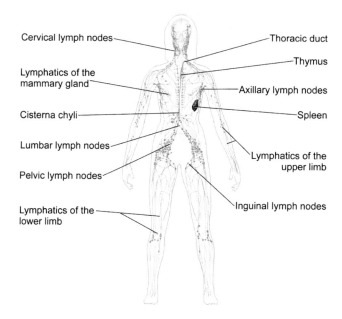

Cervical lymph nodes

Lymphatics of the mammary gland

Cisterna chyli

Lumbar lymph nodes

Pelvic lymph nodes

Lymphatics of the lower limb

Thoracic duct

Thymus

Axillary lymph nodes

Spleen

Lymphatics of the upper limb

Inguinal lymph nodes

By BruceBlaus. When using this image in external sources it can be cited as: Blausen.com staff. "Blausen gallery 2014". Wikiversity Journal of Medicine. DOI:10.15347/wjm/2014.010. ISSN 20018762. (Own work) [CC BY 3.0 (http://creativecommons.org/licenses/by/3.0)], via Wikimedia Commons

The lymphatic system is a transport system like the peripheral vascular system. However, the vessels are separate. The lymph system is composed of lymph vessels, lymph nodes, lymph ducts, and lymph nodules.

When blood is transported throughout the body, plasma from the blood flows into interstitial spaces. To prevent excess build up, the lymph system is there to drain excess fluid and plasma protein.

Lymph is collected in vessels and drains into different lymph nodes in the body where it is filtered and microbes killed. Lymph is then sent to lymph ducts which deposit it into veins to become part of the plasma in the blood supply.

Lymph is very similar to plasma in the blood. The head and neck drain into the cervical lymph nodes. The breast and upper arm are drained by the axillary lymph nodes. The hand and lower arm drain into the epitrochlear lymph nodes, and the lower extremity drains into the inguinal nodes. Lymph nodules like the thymus and spleen do not connect directly with rest of the lymph system and help protect the body from external pathogens.

References

Jarvis, C. (2008). Physical examination & health assessment (5th ed.). St. Louis, Mo.: Saunders/Elsevier.

Porth, C. (2005). Pathophysiology: Concepts of altered health states (7th ed.). Philadelphia: Lippincott Williams & Wilkins.

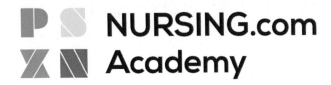
NURSING.com
Academy

One Learning Platform For Your Entire Nursing Journey

6,000+ Practice Questions	**2000+** Video Lessons	**2000+** Visual Study Tools
350+ Cheat Sheets	**150+** Nursing Care Plans	**8+** eBooks

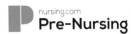
nursing.com
Pre-Nursing

Passing your HESI® or TEAS® and getting into nursing school is a breeze with the Pre-Nursing Academy.

nursing.com
Nursing Student

Courses, questions, and cheat sheets covering everything you need to learn in nursing school inside the Nursing Student Academy.

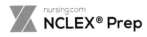
nursing.com
NCLEX® Prep

The NCLEX® Prep Academy includes NCLEX® simulation, review, questions, and study plans to help you pass with ease.

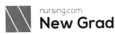
nursing.com
New Grad

Inside the New Grad Academy, you will learn to care for your patients with confidence with courses from practicing nurses.

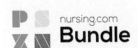
nursing.com
Bundle

2 years of access to the four NURSING.com Academies at one convenient price.

Select a plan at nursing.com

Having Trouble Finding a Brainsheet (Nursing Report Sheet) That Works?

As a gift:
Download essential templates for nursing report sheets and many more informative cheatsheets!

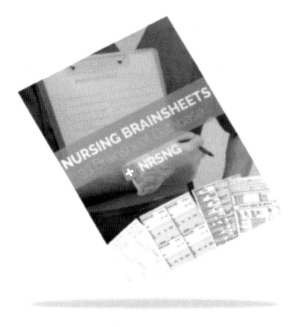

Nursing Brainsheets

Download our free PDF Brainsheet and much more!
Visit: https://nursing.com/cheat-sheets/

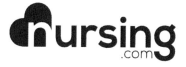

Made in the USA
Monee, IL
07 December 2023

48416248R00067